THE TRANSCENDENCE OF REIKI:

Continuing your energetic journey

Linda McCann

Nourish Your Spirit-Reiki Master Teacher

The Reiki Ideals

Just for today, I will let go of anger

Just for today, I will let go of worry.

Just for today, I will give thanks for my many blessings.

Just for today, I will do my work honestly.

Just for today, I will be kind to my neighbor and every living thing.

As presented by Mrs. Takata

ISBN : 978-1686107139
Printed in the United States of America

Special thanks go to Laurie Hamilton (Primal Painter) for the cover photo entitled "Balance within Chaos". Laurie infuses her beautiful artwork with Reiki energy for healing and to spread positive energy to the world!

Her artwork is available at: https://www.lightworkerenergyart.com

Laurie is on Facebook, Twitter and Instagram. She can be reached at Laurie-hamilton@sbcglobal.net.

Special thanks also go to Tyhson Banighen for his contribution with the Dowsing portion of the book.

Tyhson is the founder of: The Extraordinary Healing Arts Academy. You can find Tyhson hosting The Wellness Show online at https://www.facebook.com/TheExtraordinaryHealingArtsAcademy

Tyhson can be contacted at: tyhson@me.com.

The first book in this series, *The Alchemy of Reiki: Opening the door to energy work,* was awarded as a finalist in the International Book Awards, Health Category.

This book is dedicated to:

my brother Matt since without him the books wouldn't be published!

Table of Contents:

Transcending Reiki page 2

Meditation page 15

Reiki Enhancements page 18

Chakras page 28

REIKI III (Advanced) page 31

Usui Master Symbol page 33

Dai Ko Myo practice page 35

Psychic Surgery page 38

Hui Yin & Violet Breath page 43

Attunement List page 50

Reiki Master Teacher page 54

Dai Ko Mio page 56

Tibetan Fire Serpent page 60

Universal page 62

Class Outline Level I page 67

First level Reiki page 68

Class Outline Level II page 71

Second Level Reiki page 72

Class Outline Adept page 74

RMT page 76

Dowsing page 79

A Personal Message to the Reader

Welcome back! Transcending your status of apprentice at this time means you will be considered an Adept or 3rd level Reiki practitioner and from there a Reiki Master Teacher. You should be keeping an ongoing journal, learning from your practice and the practice of others. You may have been researching all the modalities to become comfortable with including them in your treatments. Daily practice including meditation should be integrated into your day to day living. Practicing on yourself, friends, family, your pets and any situations will help you expand your knowledge and gauge how effective your work is. (HUNA – effectiveness is the measure of truth). Once you have taken these classes you should work with that energy and practice until you feel comfortable enough to become a Reiki Master Teacher. Your Alchemical Reiki formulae should continue to grow as you grow in knowledge and practice. I commend you for your hard work and dedication to get to these Levels. Upon Attunements your work names you Alchemical Reiki Lightworker!

Transcending Reiki

Balance within Chaos, which is the Title of the cover painting by Laurie Hamilton (Primal Painter) is what each of us is trying to achieve when we learn Reiki and all the other modalities of energy. Your loving intent to help others is wonderful! Everyone needs help at some time in their lives. We cannot exist and be happy alone. We are all interdependent. Universal Life energy (Reiki), which we are a part of and exists all around us, is the reason we are able to use these tools.

Where are you on your spiritual path? What's your motivation leading to your decision to continue learning all you are able about Reiki and the other energy tools? Answering those questions will help you to make your decision to move forward to become a Reiki Master Teacher. The door of opportunity is opening for you to continue is this vital work. In my previous book, The Alchemy of Reiki you learned about Universal energy, Reiki and quite a few other complementary energy modalities. Once you assimilated all that information, you may complete the new classes for Adept and Master. It becomes your personal responsibility to continue your journey with your journaling, practice, meditation etc. This can be done at your own pace, remembering that you don't have to be perfect. Your sincere intentions are what matter! We are all called at different times. Try not to rush. You need to really internalize and own all you have learned.

You ultimately become responsible for your own journey, as it should be. Of course, I recommend using your RMT as a resource and gaining as much knowledge of all the "tools" you will be using in your practice. There's never going to be a "test" per se, however your knowledge will serve your purpose and you can use it as much or as little as you wish. Effectiveness is the measure of truth!

My intention for both of these books is to become workbooks for you as you are taking your classes. You may also use them to teach your own classes when you are ready. You can write your notes, symbols and perhaps begin your Alchemical Reiki formulae in these books; which will become your go-to reference. In the future, I plan to "train the trainer" so that RMT's who are so inclined might use these books in their own classes and allow this "school" to expand and share this way of practicing Reiki. A meditation CD featuring the aforementioned meditations will also become available. My sincerest wish is for these books to help you on your journey. I certainly don't know everything but, I feel that with many years of experience, I can offer what works for me in the hope it will educate you in some of the ways Reiki people think and do their work and that you will take away what you need to become an effective healer (knowing as I use that word it means Assistant).

When you hear of the word "transcendence" are you visualizing the lifting of the energy of what or whom you are working on into another realm? Can you imagine your work being transcended with energy and spirit? After you begin your personal journey on this path, and become an Adept at building your own Alchemical Reiki formulae, you certainly will have transcended any knowledge you had prior to that point. Your "Team" has entered your life to assist you in your work. In fact, you *transmuted* yourself into an ***Alchemical Reiki Lightworker!*** You are amazing! Well done!

Have you deeply considered what drives you to want to continue with this path onward to becoming a Reiki Master/Teacher? Reiki has been given by the Source to the living beings of the earth that are capable of learning and using the energy on all energy no matter what form it manifests in. Have you been practicing and researching to learn as much as you can about Reiki, the history of this modality and how some others may use it and all the applications therein? You need to have integrity and knowledge of yourself so your understanding will allow you to continue and be effective. You should have cultivated what I call "the Reiki mind" meaning that any challenge you meet -your first step in answer will be Reiki. You will be using Reiki in every situation whereby it can be the best tool possible in that situation. You will be confident that Reiki will help. You know that Reiki can never hurt anyone.

By now, you have been meditating on the symbols, becoming familiar with them, utilizing Reiki at every opportunity as you are able. You should be able to see each symbol in your mind and instantly know how to draw each one and call their name in your mind or out loud; whatever works best for you. As I indicated in my first book, The Alchemy of Reiki, a lot of the work is done in the mind so it becomes an absolute necessity to know these symbols! If not, please begin to do so. You will spend the rest of your life learning and using these energies. Always try to remain open to new ideas and ways to use what you have learned. Keep your journal as well as you can. Go back and re-read these books and your journal. You will find that you will learn something new each time. Sometimes thoughts and messages can become clearer when you look back or as more information becomes available. You get back the effort you put forth. Does that make sense to you? I would recommend taking some time for each component of Reiki.

Meditate on each symbol separately; and jot down any information you might receive. Meditate with your Angel frequently and ask for help, keeping in mind that your Angel and your Team need to be asked to step in; and you can ask for help anytime- it doesn't have to just be during meditation.. You can also meditate separately upon each Chakra and use whatever ideas pop into your mind. You can meditate with your crystals to gain a deeper knowledge whereby you learn what qualities enhance your Reiki practice. The more often you meditate, you deepen your connection to the energies you are focusing on. This in turn, opens new synapses in your brain. I also sometimes suggest drawing the symbols on paper and putting them up near your altar or on your refrigerator as a refresher. Do whatever works best for you enabling you to do this work.

As you continue on this path using Reiki I and II, you may find that you desire to go on to teach, have more energy available and 3 more symbols at your command including the Usui Master Symbol, Tibetan Master Symbol and the Tibetan Fire Serpent to "*transcend*" the work you have been doing up until this point. Adept Master level (3) and Reiki Master Teacher (4) will give you the use of three more symbols bringing your total to six. Then, I will add one of my own that I was given during a vision. I called it "Universal" and I will explain it when we come to it.

Level II is perfectly acceptable if you do not want or need to continue. Your treatment and use of the Reiki will continue to be as effective as ever. The practitioners who decide to move forward may have a Reiki business or wish to become a teacher to share all their Alchemical Reiki formulae with their students. We are all called in different ways. Whatever way you are able is the right way. I always allow my students to attend as many classes with me as they wish once they have paid and completed the level. I differ from other RMT's in this because I think the RMT should be a resource for the student and try to keep the connection also. You can become a Reiki Master without teaching. Some do not desire to teach however, they would like to acquire all the symbols and knowledge to enhance their work. An RMT should be well-versed in the history of Reiki, the usage of the symbols and have done a lot of hands-on work with the energy as I stated previously. Also, your journal should contain a synopsis, at the very least, of your work, your thoughts and your formulae. Therefore, you really should not do all the levels within a short period.

You can connect with your "Team" (which consists of spirit guides, Angels, etc.) and ask them to show or give you more information when you are ready to proceed to the Adept and Master levels. Keep in mind that you can also partner with other RMT's if you feel that might work out better for you both in running a business or class. My counsel is to use every resource that is available to you!

You have in the first book several pages of "help" for you to use while you are learning and doing Reiki. The dowsing circle, the list of steps for a Reiki treatment, disclaimer etc. are all good tools to help you determine what fits your style and your practice. In this book I also give you a step-by-step list when the time comes for you to perform an Attunement when you are at the Master level. I know that we can become overloaded with information since not only have you learned Reiki; but you have added many other modalities and concepts to that knowledge. You may have some of your own modalities to add such as a psychic gift, EFT or one of the many other tools that are out there and available to you should you care to learn about them. Many Reiki people mention "the Clairs" meaning clairaudience, clairsentience and clairvoyance. Remember you have opened new synapses in your brain. This may allow you to "see" or "hear" something about the Client you may be working on or for. Your inner self (Uni) is connected to everything; so you become more open to information intuitively. Take your time, and please don't become overwhelmed by a glut of information. I do highly recommend journaling because it may help you to develop your own insights and tricks, shortcuts or imaginative usage of all that you have learned. Journaling becomes the basis of your formulae. You need the formulae to continue on to becoming a RMT.

In order to continue on , and this may vary from RMT to RMT, I would suggest that you have at least worked with Level I and II mastering the symbols for a year at minimum; or as long as you need, practicing as much as you can. Sincerely tune in and see how you feel about it. Ask your Team. Speak to your RMT. You may be ready sooner or later than that. There is no wrong way. To be able to teach, you need a deep understanding of Reiki and of the people you will be working with. You will need to have extensive experience to be effective as a Reiki Master Teacher.

Also, in order to run a business as well; which is what you will be doing, I recommend that you pursue some classes with regard to opening and running a small business. Even if you share space at another's business; you still need to file a DBA (doing business as) and set up some type of accounting system to keep track of expenditures and income. Insurance is also an absolute requirement. This is for your protection and the Clients you are working with.

As I stated in my previous book "THE ALCHEMY OF REIKI" always have integrity in your business practices. There are many resources if you are not sure about what is needed specifically. You can also join some sites online that are exclusively for Reiki practitioners, Lightworkers, Dowsers and Empaths. Ask a question there and you will be inundated with answers. There's a lot of good information out there. However, beware as there are always negative people. Integrate the advice and knowledge that resonate with you. I am sure there are also groups supporting small businesses that can help you with any questions you may have or problems you may come across during your business life.

You have invested time and money to learn this modality. Therefore, you should charge for your treatments. I charge $25. for the initial introductory treatment. Thereafter, the charge is $45. Other RMT's (especially if they are renting space) will most likely charge $60 and upwards to $150. Also, in some states health or auto accident insurance may cover the Reiki treatment depending on what has happened with your Client. You have joined a worldwide group of dedicated practitioners who have worked hard and invested their time and money into this modality. Be proud and continue to learn and keep the integrity for all concerned in the Reiki community. Please don't compare yourself to others. We are all where we need to be. Some have been called sooner or later. Just know that you are doing what you are meant to do. I always caution my students not to judge others or yourself. We should all be united in the sincere, loving effort of helping others. We are all gifted differently. Value those differences!

Treatments for family, friends and pets come under your discretion. I certainly do not charge family or friends. Use discernment as to what works for everyone. Each situation is different and you need to figure out the best strategy for you.

Many Reiki people advocate "no free Reiki" however, that is your decision to make. Your work has value; so if you are giving it freely perhaps keep in mind that the receiver may not be appreciative of what it is you are gifting them. Be aware and if this is your "job" and you are running a business then as I said, it is up to you what, if anything you will charge. The barter system works also. You could "trade" your services for services from others. Flexibility is the key to making your Reiki business successful. Reiki is not about the money, however; there is nothing wrong with placing value on your work. Many coming to this work do so with the sincere desire to be of service to others. Many Reiki people donate their time to Hospice, nursing homes or hospitals.

Should you decide to continue, sharing your stories for Reiki becomes another teaching tool. Remember privacy and confidentiality. Perhaps you can ask permission to share a story but, not the person's name.

I have worked with those with chronic conditions such as: cancer, RA and other life changing conditions. Ideally, the person will come on an ongoing basis. If they cannot afford to do so perhaps you can work out a discount, by bartering or just gifting your services. I am an Empath so I have to fight hard to be compassionate but not invested in their disease. I am one who would save the world. We however, cannot do this. We can only work on one person at a time. It's ok to be sympathetic, understanding and focused on the person. Shield yourself with light. You can cleanse them, and shield them also. You can give holistic advice but no diagnosis or medical advice since you aren't a doctor. Always practice integrity and discernment. We must always strive to do our best in any situation whereby Reiki is being offered or practiced.

Many "own" their dis-ease and they may receive a lot of attention because of it. That in no way is meant as a judgement. Dis-ease comes from genetics, past lives, chemicals, ways of thinking or a learned behaviour... it is no easy path. Part of why they may have come to Earth at this time, could be the dis-ease is a lesson. We don't know for sure, so always try your best to be non-judgemental. When I do my "list" every morning I specify that the Reiki travel back to the beginning to release Karma, dis-ease, and anything else negative for that person. I also ask for a continuous flow of the energy until the next request. I also ask for the highest good of all, the Earth, the Angels and spirit beings who come to work with us.

My advice is to always remember not to say "my or mine" with regard to any condition of the body unless it is a positive statement. Your inner self (Uni) will take that as law. Our inner self is comparable to a 7 year old child-very literal.

This will probably always be an on-going conscious effort on your part. If you slip, just go forward and try to do better. I find myself doing this occasionally and I immediately correct myself. Don't "own" the dis-ease!

I also "teach" my Clients. I share meditations with them. I also talk about not owning the dis-ease and give them ideas that may have worked for me or other Clients.

If someone has a chronic condition; you can do a Healing Attunement (discussed later) which will open them to more energy. I also send Reiki on a continuous flow and ask that their "Team" also receive a continuous flow to share as needed. As I mentioned previously, I have a list and I try to add as many names as I comfortably can to receive Reiki on an on-going basis. I also send it to the past, present & future with the HSZSN. I send it to multiple timelines, known or unknown realities. You can't change the past, however you can hope to eliminate the emotion or pain and take the lesson to move forward.

I also find that those of us who do this work usually attract those conditions that we are familiar with. That makes sense to me because at the very least, you are familiar and empathetic to what your Client is experiencing.

I recently read of a scientific experiment using mouse cancer cells and they were given Reiki which caused them to change for the better! How amazing is that? I am really very excited whenever we get some validation for the work we do. In our society, ***stress*** leads to many uncomfortable situations including dis-ease.

Many people who come for Reiki seem to be the type A personality and that makes sense to me. They are all working hard in every way to take care of themselves, their families, their homes and their jobs. By taking the hour to have a Reiki treatment they are facilitating their own release of stress. During the time they are with the Reiki practitioner they are probably being given some insight and direction as to how they can ease these situations. Any insights that come to you while they are with you should be shared in a manner that will be comfortable for them. Self-care is vitally important for the Reiki practitioner and each Client. I talk about this during intake because many women especially are conditioned to give to others and feel guilty if they receive. You can't drive your car without gas so therefore it makes sense that you need to take care of your vehicle (your body) in a similar manner.

Meditation

The first suggestion I have for you would be to "step into" whatever you are meditating on. For instance if you start with Cho-Ku-Rei, then I suggest getting yourself ready by being seated, closing your eyes, putting your fingers against your thumb (indicates to your Uni that you are going to meditate), deep breathing and See, Say and draw the symbol in the air or in your mind. Visualize yourself or just knowing it is you stepping into the symbol treating it as if it can communicate, which it will. Act "as if" and it will happen for you. Prepare yourself ahead of time by making a list of questions you might like to ask. I think you will be surprised at the information you may get from each thing that you meditate on. Journal whatever information you get. This will become a habit the more you do so. You can also do this more than once as your knowledge deepens and you may have further questions or need further insights. Have fun with it also!

Another suggestion for your meditation sessions would be to do it as you have done before. You can (in your mind or physically) go to a place that is sacred and comfortable to you. I have a designated area outside centered near a fountain and a circular patio to represent the spiral of the Cho-Ku-Rei. I use this space for myself and in my classes during the nicer months. Once there in your sacred space (in your mind or in person), you can ask to be shown the symbol, crystal or Angel or whatever you are working on to see if there's any information for you. I find there is always more knowledge to be gained. Now, I know that we are all busy these days however, you can do these meditations briefly and still get some insights. If you are new to meditation just do the best you can. If you go to a Reiki share perhaps all concerned would be willing to be led in a meditation on a particular aspect of the Reiki energy. Practice makes perfect!

You can also ask your RMT to help you with some sort of daily practice which will become really advantageous to you and your Reiki. I mentioned in my last book that I do Reiki while I am in the shower as well as throughout my day. I have a list I work on every day. The more you use the energies the more "flow" comes through you. If you don't do well at visualizing, you can write out whatever it is that you wish to work on. Place it on your altar, your refrigerator, your vision board or wherever it is that you work on your goals. You can use the Antakharana and make a Reiki grid. This will be explained a little further on which allows you to use some new tools for your work.

Note: A version of the Antakharana was used by Hitler for the Nazis. The symbol itself has no allegiance to anything or anyone. It is just that: a sacred symbol that he had no right to use for the horrific tragedies that he perpetuated. I had some trouble with it in the beginning because of that association, however it is only a symbol and it is a connection to the sacred. Use your own best judgement as to what you are comfortable using. Hitler was into Occult knowledge and misused that information to perpetuate evil with his work. We always try to do the work – In the Light.

REIKI ENHANCEMENTS

On the Reiki grid place a Master crystal in the center of the paper or cloth Antakharana. Then you may place six quartz crystals or other crystals you may be drawn to use, facing inwards focusing their energies on the Master crystal. Quartz, Apopholite, Selenite and Herkimer diamonds are all usable in this context because they enhance the energy of the Master crystal. My Master crystal is quartz, yours might be something else. Place your written intention on the grid, or a picture of whom or what you are working on or for. Using this grid also allows you to have a continuous flow to that Client. When I do my "list" in the morning, I also ask that the Reiki be sent on a continuous flow as needed. I send it to the Source, the Angels and Guides for their usage and to share with whomever they work with. You can send to a specific time, place or all of the aforementioned. I also would "charge" the grid with all the symbols I have at my command. We know from HUNA (Hawaiian philosophy) that energy flows where attention goes. Focusing on whatever it is that you are trying to manifest will indicate to the energies that you wish to accomplish your goal through your intention and work. You can lay down the large piece of paper or cloth with the Antakharana and place crystals facing towards the center where you have put your master crystal.

For the grid, a flat piece of paper printed with the Antakharana can be placed on your altar, and you may put a written goal or a picture in the center on top of your master crystal. You would then clear your mind, have the intention of a continuous flow of Reiki to whatever it is you are working on. Do all of your symbols and try to visualize in your mind what outcome you would like although I prefer to ask for an unlimited outcome. I choose not to put limitations on anything because I positively do not know all that is available for whatever it is I am asking for. There are no limits is another HUNA thought so in this way, you may decide to leave that open for interpretation by your Team and the Reiki energies. There are stores online that you can purchase cloth printed with the Antakharana to work with instead of a piece of paper. If you are an artist you could also draw this symbol and use it. Either way your usage of the symbols combined with your intent will create the vibration that will attract the energies. You can also get a copy and print from internet. I have included a picture of the Antakharana on the next page.

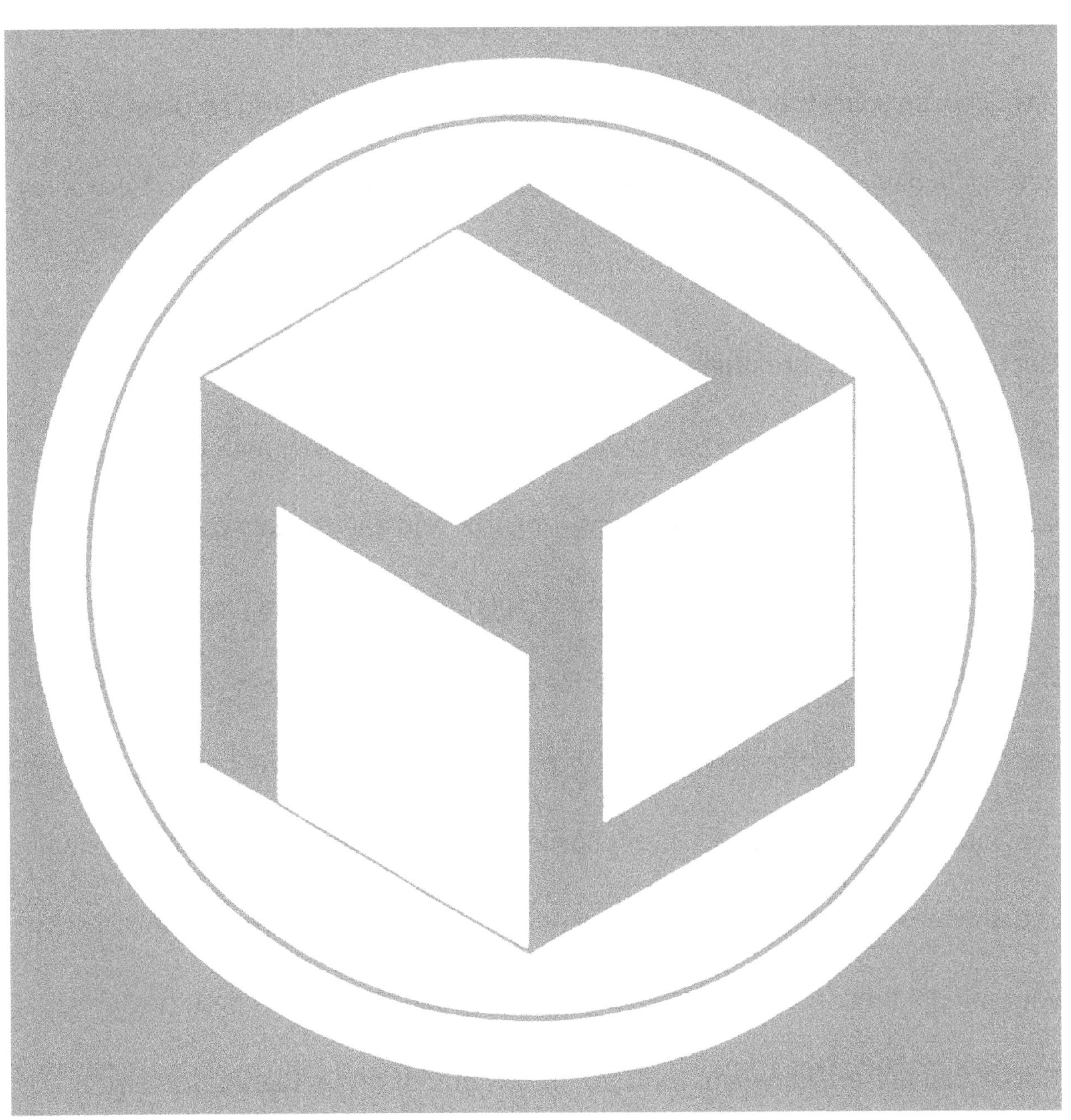

Also, whilst meditating you can hold crystals in your hands or place them around you or on your body. You may choose them based on their properties or you may have chosen some that you have meditated with and connected to. I am all about getting "a bang for my buck" meaning that in this case more is better! Here is my meditation to meet your Reiki guides:

Get yourself ready, breathing deeply and settling yourself down into whatever you are sitting or lying on. You could use the Antakharana symbol to make the connection to your guide(s) by placing it nearby and any crystals you may be guided to use. By breathing slowly and deeply you can create a picture in your mind of your sacred space while clearing all other thoughts from your mind. You are continuing to settle down and your body and limbs may feel heavier. Picture the Antakharana somewhere in this space. Focus on what you see, hear or smell. You are very relaxed and comfortable. Visualizing the Antakharana symbol; ask in your mind if there are any guide(s) that want to step forth and connect with you. Not all Being(s) are known to us. Give this a moment remembering you are picturing this all in your mind. A Being(s) will come. You may greet the Being and ask for their oversight and direction in your life and with your Reiki work. The

Being may speak to you directly, give you a token or both. If you are not familiar with this Being you may ask for a name if they haven't given it to you in the initial contact. Express your gratitude that they are willing to work with you. Keep breathing, when you feel enough information has been shared- slowly become aware of your surroundings, when you are ready, open your eyes. Please do journal all the information you can remember. This will allow you to research this Being and perhaps get some insight into the token or whatever they have said to you. If the token or gift is something you can purchase, I would buy it and place it on my altar to remind me of the information that I was given. You always have a "Team" that works with you. They can come and go. When you are doing Reiki- being a human, you may have forgotten a step, however the "Team" will step in and assist you. I have had Clients say they felt other presences and hands on their body whilst they were receiving a treatment. As I said in my previous book "THE ALCHEMY OF REIKI", there are myriad different positive energies that surround you and will work with you. All of this is a wonderful gift to us on our journey to serve as an ***Alchemical Reiki Lightworker***!

I have recently been given another way to meet your Guides because I have learned that some do not have a special place that they would go to whilst meditating. You would get yourself ready by following the aforementioned steps for Meditation. Clear your mind and then visualize yourself in the dark facing forward. As you begin slowly walking (picturing this in your mind), you will see the outline of light gleaming from around a door. Remember to keep breathing slowly and deeply. Continue to walk towards the door knowing that you are safe and will be entering a safe place. The light is golden and welcoming even though you are only seeing the outline. You go to the door and open it. You walk through into the area beyond. The light is soft and welcoming- you feel and are completely safe. Ask in your mind if a Guide is there for you. What are you seeing? A being or beings will step forward. You will be given a name and at this point, you may ask any questions you might have. Perhaps they will say something or give you a gift. You will remember what they look like, their name and whatever they say or do. When you feel you have spent sufficient time- thank your Guide(s) and go back through the door. Remember you are breathing slowly and deeply, however you are starting to become aware of your physical presence. Allow yourself to slowly "come back" to your physical body. Open your eyes. Write down any information you have gotten. You may not recognize the name of the Being(s) so take some time to research as you are able. Think about what they may have said and what the gift (if any) means to you. Often we get a guide that there is no recorded information for. You can still trust this information because there are many spirit beings working with us. This Being may be someone like us who has ascended to do this work on the other side. You can ask them directly while you are in the midst of the meditation if you so desire. There are many ways to meditate so these are a couple of examples to help you during your own practice of meditation initially. You will find what works best for you.

You may want to do these meditations a few times until you feel comfortable with the information that you have been given.

Come back to your notes regarding your various meditations especially if you did not understand easily what was said or happened. The light will become brighter in your mind as you are focusing on it and perhaps by researching what was said or gifted. Remember our HUNA thought: Energy flows where attention goes. Also, there are many meditations available from various sources online if you would feel better having someone else guide you.

I faithfully use "The Secret" meditation because it allows me to relax and focus on great energy when I am trying to get to sleep. The subliminal messages carryover into my daily life and they are much appreciated. We always need to be working on ourselves, our mind and spirit. Meditation allows these positive messages to become deeply ingrained in our subconscious (Uni) and will become second nature whereby we utilize all we have heard and learned. Sometimes life can seem overwhelming and negative. My motto is: This too shall pass. If things aren't great at the moment, just remember life can change in the blink of your eye. Focus on the good in your life and know that you are worthy to have a happy life. Trust and whatever you desire will come to you.

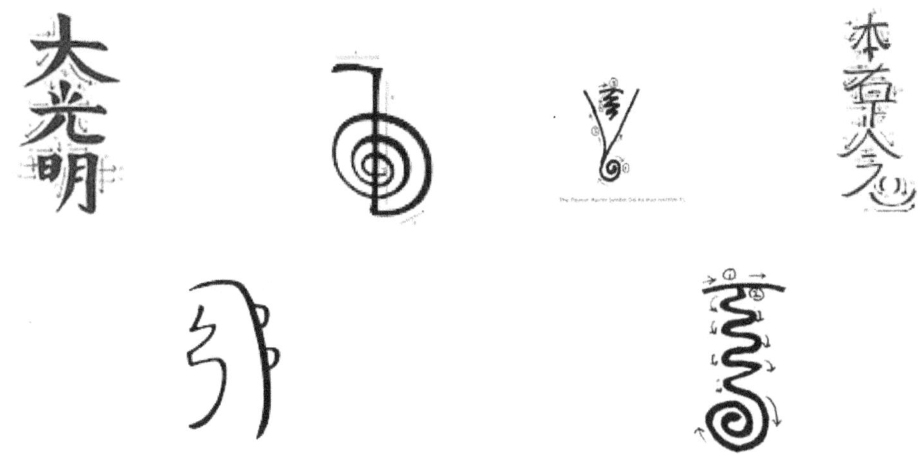

THE REIKI BOX

The Reiki box can be any box that you may have on hand or you can purchase one online from a variety of stores. You can write down goals, intentions, desires etc. on a piece of paper and I personally, would draw the symbols on the piece of paper to put inside also, although it is not a requirement. Once the paper or papers has been put into the box, close it and get ready to do Reiki. Place your hands on the box, focus your intention on the written request and of course, draw all your symbols over the box. You may place crystals inside and outside. I would send the Reiki on a continuous flow. If you have time, you could do this daily or as often as you are able. You can also request your "Team" to send Reiki to this goal. This is an easy way, especially in our busy world, to have a focused intent to manifest whatever it is that you desire. The aforementioned are all tools you can incorporate into your Reiki practice or not. How you do your work is totally up to you. It is imperative that you develop your formulae and your practice. You will benefit and also your Clients will benefit from added enhancements.

Shamanistic thought allows you to step out of Time and Space. So, too does the Reiki symbol of HSZSN allow you to do the same. There are other planes of existence and other levels of Spirit. As you do your work as a RMT you will grow into transcending knowledge and perhaps incorporate the ideas of multiple dimensions, known or unknown realities and of course, past, present and future.

The energy is a free gift from the Source once you learn the application of intent, use of the symbols and practice. Come to this work with an open mind and heart and you will be astounded at what you can accomplish!

CHAKRAS

We learned about the Chakra system from "The Alchemy of Reiki". There are many books on this subject should you care to deepen your knowledge. There are a total of 16 Chakras. I have already covered the 7 that people know about in my first book. There are also Chakras in each hand and foot which should never be excluded during a treatment. What most people may not be aware of is that there are 5 Chakras over and above the Crown Chakra. They are as follows:

- Seafoam green is 8th above the Crown-Center of Divine Love, spiritual skills
- Blue green is the 9th – Soul blue print & total skills from all Lifetimes
- Pearl White is the 10th - Divine creativity
- Pink-orange is the 11th- Advanced spiritual teleportation, telekinesis
- Shining Gold is the 12th-Cosmos connection to Divinity

I mention these so you become aware of them. You can imagine them in your mind and use your pendulum to dowse them if you feel the need. A Client may have a past life issue or want to become open to working on the etheric plane.

Most likely you will not do much work with these until you are quite far along on your path. You need a good solid foundation to work with these energies. Again, research and learn. If you do decide to try working with these, please do ask your Team and their Team to shield you both from any misjudgments or mistakes since you are not fully aware of what you are doing. What do I mean by that? I myself have been doing this work for many years and I hesitate to delve into energies I don't know a lot about. If I chose to do some work with these Chakras I would do as much research as possible and also ask my Team to facilitate and shield me. It is important to be grounded, shielded and surrounded by Light because it has been known that when you are emitting a bright Light, dark entities may come to take an interest. You never want to open the door to anything negative. You can use your pendulum to clear and shield also. We are always clearing because certain places are a hotbed of energy such as: hospitals and nursing homes, just to name a couple. A lot of people have died or been in pain in those places and sometimes there is a residue of energy from either not crossing over or the angst of the pain they suffered. Anytime I go to these types of places I shield myself and clear when I am out of there. I send Reiki to the entire place and I also send souls over if that is required. You will become more intuitive as you work to move forward on your path to the Light. If you don't notice any of these things don't worry about it. I just wanted you to be aware that there are many things in this world that we don't see or aren't aware of. Also, when removing anything please fill the empty space with love. Nature abhors a vacuum.

You should be aware also that some people are energy vampires whether they do so purposely or unknowingly. Shield yourself. You can try to clear them with the pendulum and then ask that they be shielded in light. Don't be surprised if it doesn't work. These types of people for whatever reason require lots of attention and seem to want to take others' energy and give nothing back. Do the best you can and if you have to, limit your contact with them. You will know them by how drained you seem to feel after you have been in contact with them. This happens to all of us occasionally but if it becomes a problem then you need to step away. This comes under the heading of "self-care".

REIKI III ADVANCED

You will find when you are ready for this level that your class may consist of only you or perhaps another person or two. Many Reiki people do not continue on because, as I said the Level I and II allow you to do anything your mind can imagine. Your Master Teacher may have other people available to come for a treatment during class and they may share their own experiences and knowledge.

Groups are great because the energy is magnified. Group Reiki is really amazing! I have some Clients who prefer to have this form because the energies are so strong. Imagine if you will, a group of four or more people working on you! You will get off that table feeling like a million bucks! Group Reiki is very effective for chronic conditions.

In this class you will learn about the Antakharana and ways to use that symbol. This symbol is already printed on a piece of paper. You do not normally draw it or follow the procedures that are vital for the other symbol usage. I carry one in my purse, have one under my bed and others in my Reiki areas. You do not have to have an attunement to use this symbol. All other symbols require attunement given by RMT to the student. This is the "bridge to the sacred" symbol. This symbol comes from India and Tibet. We also use it in the USA as part of our Reiki practice. Antakharana translated means interior mind which we know from HUNA as being the Unihipili-subconscious mind. Uni is responsible for all bodily processes and connection to all that is. Using Antakharana allows Uni to access energy specifically for the "interior mind" and tap into collective consciousness. This is where "intuition" resides. You can develop intuition and knowing by being open to it. I am sure you have had "gut" feelings before. You need to learn to trust those feelings because Uni picks up information on a subliminal level.

Once you are attuned on any level, it is up to you to focus on your own research, meditation and practice. You will get out of this what you put into it. Does that make sense to you? Reiki is a lifelong study. There is always new information and new modalities to add. There are many schools out there that use the basic Reiki but may have their own specific focus. Many teachers have also been inspired and teach new symbols as they grow into the light of Reiki. I myself was fortunate to receive one such symbol which I spoke of earlier in the book called Universal. This symbol will be explained later on in this book.

USUI MASTER SYMBOL

You will also get another symbol which is called the Usui Master Symbol. This symbol will help in opening a channel for more energy from the Source. It is a very powerful symbol. This symbol enhances your usage of the others. It is similar to having your faucet wide open. This symbol is great to use for your meditation practice as it will help open you to more energy. This symbol allows you to physically connect to your higher self (Aumaukua) and from there to the source. The Usui Master symbol allows you to amplify the energies. I have heard it described as more powerful than the three first symbols combined.

If you remember from my first book, I mentioned that you should use the symbols in the order they were taught and learned by you. Now that you have been attuned for this Usui Master symbol, I recommend using it first as this symbol will amplify the energies of Cho-Ku-Rei, Sei-Hei-Ki, Hon-Sha-Ze-Sho-Nen. Again, I reiterate you should use all your symbols all the time! Your experiences using the Reiki and all other modalities that you add will help you make this symbol your own and add it to your ***Alchemical Reiki formulae.*** Previously, I remind you that we are always a work in progress and our Reiki practice should always be evolving as you add enhancements. My belief is the more you can do for your Client; the more territory you cover. You may not know at what level the work you are doing is affecting your Client, but you can be confident that you are using the best of your abilities and knowledge. Your Client will surely appreciate this! Remember also, if you get busy and drawn away from doing Reiki every day, the symbols always remain in your Aura. They are with you for life. Therefore, you can step back into doing Reiki again anytime. I would suggest getting Attuned again though however, if you aren't in contact with a RMT then the Reiki will come back the more you are using it.

I truly believe that we all should be Attuned as many times as possible. Why? I mentioned previously that Reiki opens new synapses in our brain, so it makes sense to me, that the more you receive the Attunements; you will open the channels for more flow of energy- which becomes our goal.

The Usui Master Symbol – Dai Ko Myo is the master symbol that Dr. Usui used. This symbol is very powerful, combining the power of the previous three: CKR, SHK and HSZSN. The focus is transformation or transcendence at the spiritual level. This is only used by RMT's. My rule is: all symbols all the time. Even though this covers the first three, there is no harm in doing all your symbols and much benefit can be derived. I have seen some RMT's double up symbols. They draw each symbol with both hands at the same time. There are no limits (HUNA) and this may serve well especially in those tough cases. We must remain fluid. The time involved is minimal and by using all your symbols all the time, you will become the **Alchemical Reiki Lightworker** you wish to be. Remember to see, say and draw each symbol. You are training yourself to be able to instantly call this symbol to mind visually. I only have to think "Reiki" and the energy comes flowing through my hand chakras. Occasionally, in public the energy will flow and I know that someone needs it even though I probably don't know who that may be. This may happen when you truly become the "channel".

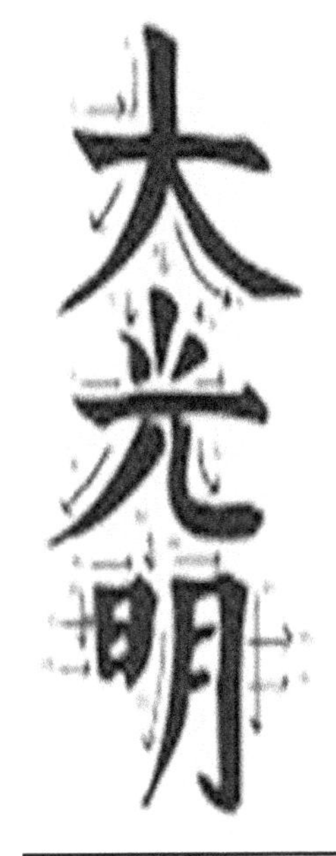

DAI KO MIO-Usui Master Symbol

DAI KO MYO

(This page left blank for your practice)

PSYCHIC SURGERY

This can also be called Aura clearing and William Lee Rand, (International Ctr. for Reiki Training - ICRT) developed the technique based on what he had learned from a Hawaiian Kahuna while he was living there. A Kahuna is an Alchemist in broad terms because they use the precepts from HUNA and other knowledge to "heal" and they have their own formulae. In Reiki, we step outside of Time and Space as do Shamans and Kahunas.

This Aura clearing "surgery" can be used to release blockages which you would determine by asking the Client to "tune-in" and ask their inner child where the blockage is occurring and if they would be willing to release it? If the Client wants to share the information that is fine however, they do not need to disclose what they want to work on or exactly what the blockage may be. The Client may have a chronic dis-ease and in order to release it they would need your help to let it go. Keep in mind that if this is a situation whereby the person has had that disease for years, it may take many sessions to release it. In some cases, it may not be released at all. Do your best however, you cannot control a persons' thinking or subliminal reluctance to release a blockage. This is one reason why my advice is never to "own" the dis-ease by saying "my (condition)" or anything similar. This is good advice for you to share with your client. It requires a retraining of our thinking and constant vigilance. While the Client is tuning in by doing this, you could be doing a Reiki treatment. When the Client is ready it may help to question them as to where the blockage is located, what it may look like etc. You also may have "felt" it when you scanned the Aura or dowsed the Chakras. Everyone gets blocked at some time or another because we are all exposed to negative energy. Please do note that never are you to diagnose or claim to "heal" in our world. As I said in my last book, the work we do facilitates the body to kick in with its own healing. A lot of blockages can come from the way we think. Our environment, past lives and genetics can all contribute to the blockage. Also, remember the "big picture", as this may be the path that this soul has chosen. We can only do our best and release to the highest good of all concerned. It may be that the Client needs time to consider the blockage and be willing to release it. We can get comfortable with "dis-ease" because it is something we know and are familiar with on a daily basis. Releasing it could bring about major life changes and some are not willing to do this. This is a sad scenario, but true. That choice is totally up to the Client.

How would we go about doing this "psychic surgery"? You would draw the Usui Master Symbol on each hand, of course repeating the name three times whilst clapping your hands. Do the same with the Cho Ku Rei and then also draw the power symbol (CKR) down the front of your body for protection. Draw CKR over each chakra to empower them. You can ask both of your "Teams" to participate and say a prayer if you wish. Your intention should be that this will be a powerful release for your Client. It can become quite emotional. Mentally tune in and I do HUNA breathing prior to doing anything with a Client. You would breathe in deeply and release the breath with a HA! sound. Do this four times. This will build MANA (power or energy). Each breath honors something- subconscious (Uni), conscious (Uhane), superconscious (Aumakua), and the Source. Your focus should be intent and I would ask for a continuous clearing until the dis-ease is gone. Confidence is a key component for you as the practitioner. Also, I would ask that the "clearing" go back to the beginning of time, now and forward to the future, multidimensional levels known or unknown realities. Remember there are no limits (Huna) and this covers all the bases.

I would visualize my fingers extending and able to reach inside the body where the Client has indicated the blockage. Pull the blockage out and send this energy to the Violet flame of St. Germain and to the white light to be disbursed for all time. Also, visualize the empty space as being filled with healing, reiki and light. Will this work? As I said previously, this can depend on a myriad of factors.

The surgery can't physically hurt your Client although it may bring up emotional issues. At the very least, we hope the procedure may initiate their desire to be rid of the blockage. You may have to do this more than once. Do encourage them to keep up with their regular visits to their Doctor also. In the case of cancer, you could do this surgery for a tumor if you know the location. Once you feel that you are finished with the surgery visualize your fingers becoming their original shape. Fill the empty space with Reiki and love. I would also ask Archangel Raphael to fill the Client with his green light of healing. If you work with other specific Beings then by all means, use whatever you think might help this Client.

This probably won't be something you will do often unless you are dealing with Clients that are coming specifically for this reason. They may have been referred to you or if you are working in a hospital setting you might want to employ this method. I would also use a "healing attunement" in the case of a chronic

Dis-ease. Discuss the attunement with the Client and you would do a Level I attunement for them prior to the treatment. Thereafter, they will be attuned and the energy will be magnified. There are a lot of ways to expand your knowledge and treatment capabilities with these new tools. Step out in faith, that you as the

Alchemical Reiki Lightworker will be guided to always do the right thing for your Clients and yourself.

THE HUI YIN AND THE VIOLET BREATH

We learn about these two practices prior to learning how to give an attunement (Reiju-spirit of the source) to our students. Most likely if you are taking Advanced or Adept Reiki, you will be continuing on to Reiki Master Teacher. Dr. Usui did not teach this practice. He gifted his students with Reiju and no touching or symbols were used. I believe that this practice of the Violet breath and the Hui Yin came from another Reiki school. I know that many of the Western Reiki practitioners and the International Center for Reiki Training use these methods to attune their students. I also use them to attune my students or to give a healing attunement in cases of severe or chronic illness because that is the way I was taught and I believe that they work to allow the maximum amount of energy.

The Master Level information will describe step by step how to prepare for and give an attunement. Remembering to practice, practice and more practice!

THE HUI YIN

The Hui Yin is the area located between your genitals and anus – the perineum area. As the RMT, you would contract this area similar to doing a "Kegel" exercise although in this instance, you would keep it contracted for as long as you are giving the attunement. This can be difficult. Doing this daily will enable you to do this as you strengthen the muscles. This practice holds the Chakra energy in your body while you are "gifting" the Reiju (attunement).However, some schools do not do these practices to give the attunement. I am not quite sure how they do their attunements or initiation, but this is the way I learned and the way I teach. I have read that this is a Western version of Attunement. It really doesn't matter because this is what you will learn and how you will proceed to use it. It all comes down to intention. The ritual of the Attunement becomes the channel for the gift of Reiki to your student. Your intention and Your Team convey this "gift" via the ritual that you will learn and use.

THE VIOLET BREATH

You may know that the violet flame comes from St. Germain who is an Ascended Master Alchemist. It is my belief that the Violet breath originated from that flame which is sacred fire of higher dimensions. This violet flame transmutes negativity into Light. I directly work with St. Germain in the same manner as my other spirit guides. The technique whereby you are using the Violet Breath combines with the technique of Hui Yin to create the attunement energy needed to "gift" the student with the symbols and level of Reiki that they are learning. You would contract the Hui Yin and do the Violet Breath at the same time. Draw in a breath, place your tongue to the roof of your mouth behind the top teeth and visualize your breath as a violet light coming down through your crown chakra, flowing through your tongue, down the front of your body through the Hui Yin (which is still contracted) and up the spine to the center of your head. Holding your tongue in this position also holds in the energy from the Crown and Root Chakra completing the closed containment of the energy.

Your student will be seated, their eyes closed and hands in prayer position. You may have incense, candles, music or have used a Tibetan singing bowl or music to "set" the atmosphere prior to the attunement. How elaborate is up to how much time you have to devote to your set up. Our Uni (inner child) loves ritual! By making a ritual of the gifting, our inner selves (Uni) will remember and view the gifting as sacred. The Reiju opens the door for the student to become the channel for this energy. Levels must be given one at a time in my experience. Thus, in order to continue to this Adept or third level, you must have had first and second level attunements. You cannot give the attunement to yourself.

I also set up my sacred space to give the Reiju. I clear it with all my symbols, light candles or incense, and perhaps place flowers to gift to the student after the attunement along with their Certificate of level completion. I use the singing bowl also to clear energies; then I usually have some type of new age music playing. I place a chair in the center of the room for the student to sit. Previously I would have instructed the student that when it is their turn, they come into the room quietly and sit, closing their eyes and placing their hands in the prayer position. I advise them to keep their eyes closed and there is to be no talking throughout the ritual. I will also have asked both Teams to attend and help with this ritual.

Having prepared yourself by doing the Violet breath and contracting the Hui yin, you will place your hands on your students' head and close your eyes as they will have theirs closed throughout this reiju process. You will have the intention to "connect" with the person. Visualizing and drawing the Tibetan Fire Serpent over the Crown Chakra begins this process. Placing your hands on top of their head, meditate briefly to connect. Exhale into the Crown Chakra (Dai Ko Myo) the Tibetan Master Symbol (Dai Ko Mio), drawing the Usui Master symbol over the Crown you would guide this with your hand after drawing it down to the base of the skull. Then Sei Hei Ki will be drawn over the head, moving into the crown, guiding with your hand to the base of the skull. We would continue with the Hon Sha Ze Sho Nen in the same way. Continuing by touching the students left shoulder, lifting their hands still in prayer position on top of their head and drawing the Cho-Ku-Rei. Try not to lose the contact of touch while you walk around the front bringing down the hands and opening them in a cupped position. I keep a hand on their shoulder. Draw the Cho-Ku-Rei and lightly slap their hands 3X. Walk around the back with your hands on their shoulders looking with your inner eye into the Crown-picturing a red ball of fire-saying to yourself "you are a successful Reiki healer" and repeat 3X with intention of acceptance by the subconscious (Uni) mind of the student. Bringing your hands to the base of the skull, visualize a door with the power symbol and say "I now seal this process with Divine love & wisdom". Picture the door being closed and locked. Intend the student to be directly connected to the Reiki Source. Move to the front, hold hands at waist level with palms facing student. Inhale, then exhale up and down their front releasing the Hui Yin and Violet Breath. Ask the student to breathe deeply and open their eyes. Congratulate them and give them their Certificate and/or flower. This is a Level I attunement. You could practice with a doll or stuffed animal to get yourself used to the "flow" having your list with you as a resource step-by-step. There is nothing wrong with having your list by your side to remind yourself of each step. We don't often do the RMT class and it serves my purpose to have this sheet available for reference.

For Level II you would add Sei Hei Ki and Hon Sha Ze Sho Nen to the drawing of the symbols over their hands. For Adept (third level or Advanced) you would add the Dai Ko Myo and for RMT you would add the Dai Ko Mio, Tibetan Fire Serpent and Universal. I know it sounds complicated so that is why I made you a chart to follow. You can fill in with pictures of symbols so you can see it at a glance. Once you have contracted the Hui Yin and have done the Violet breath, you will want to move right along because it is difficult to hold for a long time.

As I say that, I don't want you to get too caught up thinking you're going to make a mistake. You may but, just know that your Guides and Angels are with you, helping you do this Attunement. If you forget to hold Violet Breath and contract Hui Yin just do it quickly again. You do not have to start over with the Attunement just keep going. Your Team will step up and fill in.

Don't worry that you will forget how to do this. Later in the book I will give you a list that you can follow as you are doing the Attunement. Your teacher should also have showed you exactly how and what to do. Once you have practiced it a few times, it will get easier to remember, noting that you will not be giving any attunements until you are at Master Level. You may have to wait for some years to bring a student to Reiki Master Teacher. Your students need to really be experienced and able to become a teacher. This is not something that should be done in a day. As a RMT, you should be a Mentor for your students, working with them if their goal is to move forward into becoming an RMT. If possible, have the student attend some of your classes thereby getting an idea what is involved in teaching and materials that may be needed.

THE ATTUNEMENT (REIJU)

(Draw the required symbols in the margin)

1. Have student come to the place you have set aside to do the attunement, having prepared prior with music, candles etc. Student will sit, close eyes and place hands in prayer form.
2. You will close your eyes, take the Violet breath and contract Hui Yin. Place your hands on the head lightly drawing the Tibetan Fire Serpent from top of head to base of spine.
3. Visualizing the Tibetan Master Symbol (Dai Ko Mio) and using your hand guide from top to bottom while exhaling into the Crown.
4. Draw Usui Master Symbol (Dai Ko Myo) over Crown and picture it moving into the Crown guiding with your hand.
5. Draw Hon Sha Ze Sho Nen, picturing it moving and being guided by your hand into the Crown.
6. Touch their left shoulder, lift hands-draw Cho Ku Rei, keeping your hand on their should walk around in front lowering their hands to an open cupped position, draw the Cho Ku Rei again and lightly slap their palms 3X knowing that the Cho Ku Rei is being placed in their aura.
7. Walk back around keeping connection, put your hands on their shoulders visualizing a red ball of fire-saying (in your mind) "You are a successful Reiki healer" repeating 3X intending acceptance by their subconscious mind.
8. Bring your hands to the base of the skull. Say (in your mind) "I now seal this process with Divine love & wisdom" picturing a door with the power symbol being closed/locked. Intend student to be directly connected to the Reiki Source.
9. Move to the front hold your hands at waist level palms facing student, inhale, then exhale up and down while releasing Hui Yin.
10. Ask student to breathe deeply and open their eyes with your Congratulations on being Level I.
11. Level II you would add Sei Hei Ki and Hon Sha Ze Sho Nen at step number 6 for Level II.
12. Adept-Master level you would add DKM.
13. Reiki Master Teacher you would add DKM & Universal.

Ok so there you are! You have done your first Attunement. You can also Attune Clients for healing purposes or do the Violet Breath by breathing it to surround them with healing. Archangel Raphael also can help if asked as he is in charge of healing. His color is green. You can surround your Client with the breath and any Angelic colors that you think may help. This is effective for chronic disease, abuse issues etc. The Attunement opens them to more energy. I also always have the intention that the Reiki flows on a continuous basis. Our Team comes in to play for this aspect. I send Reiki to the Source (or whatever you choose to call it), all Spirit Beings that work for the highest good of all, Mother Earth and all that dwell therein. Then I get specific with my list adding situations and all concerned, specific people who may have asked for remote healing or to their Angels to disperse on an as needed basis, family, friends, pets and you could continue on and on.

Another way to do Remote healing is to visualize the person you wish to work on, psychically calling their spirit body with the intent for healing and picturing in your mind working on them and going through the process of a treatment although you would only spend about thirty seconds to a minute on each area. When you feel the treatment is complete you would release the spirit back to the physical body and release your connection to them in your own mind. You could also place a picture of whom or what you want to do some work for, on your Reiki grid, box or your altar. Writing down your goals in your personal handwriting alerts the Universe to your intention of manifesting these goals. Focusing on your goals will indeed bring manifestation of your dreams and/or the dreams of your Clients.

I always have something I am working on. My altar is set up with Antakharana and crystals, perhaps a picture of someone, or a written "check" for unlimited prosperity. Those are just a few examples of what you can use your altar for to focus on your desires.

A cloth as a base in a color that you prefer, the Antakhrana, a grid or box -then your focus (which can be a person, place or thing), and then placing crystals to enhance your work. I also keep a pendulum there to do clearing and other dowsing to add to my work. I would then do all my symbols and these can be written and placed there on the altar also, with the intention of manifesting whatever it is that you wish to do. I would also draw the symbols in the air over the altar with the intent of continuous flow. I also place pictures of whom or what

I may be working on, written desires for instance: unlimited health, unlimited wealth etc. Use your imagination and what matters to you most. When you feel something has been completed that you are working on-take it off or out of the altar, box or grid. You can place something new anytime you feel the need. Give some attention to this every single day. You may be surprised what happens for you.

REIKI MASTER TEACHER

This part of your journey, should you decide to advance requires a good working knowledge of Reiki. Also, I would encourage a daily practice which will help you to become as familiar with it as you are with yourself. You will need to have completed Reiki I, II, and Advanced. I suggest you give yourself time to digest each level and do as much work as you can. A Reiki Master Teacher should have a daily practice of working with the energy. The state of our world and humanity itself requires much work to be done on a daily and ongoing basis. This is the *Chemickal Marriage which was the ultimate goal of the Alchemist,* so to speak. The Alchemist was practicing his/her formulae over the years with the intention of achieving this marriage which transcended the materials used from the beginning. The Alchemist was combining Intellect, intention, knowledge and spirit. The Alchemist was a combination of scientist and in some peoples' thinking he/she was a magician. You too, will culminate your work in a "marriage" of intention, practice and observation. The RMT is the result of the marriage becoming complete. You are never done learning, however at this point when you become the Master you should have the ability to teach what you have learned and your focus may move from Clients to students. I try to do some of each. It is good practice to keep your connection to Clients as well as students.

The more you practice the better the flow. Reiki is an extremely powerful tool!It is analogous to using your muscles. You know the more you use them the stronger they become. It is the same with Reiki.

DAI KO MYO (Tibetan Master Symbol)

This symbol heals at the Soul level while the other Usui symbols heal Aura and the physical. This page left blank for your own practice.

Di Ko Mio

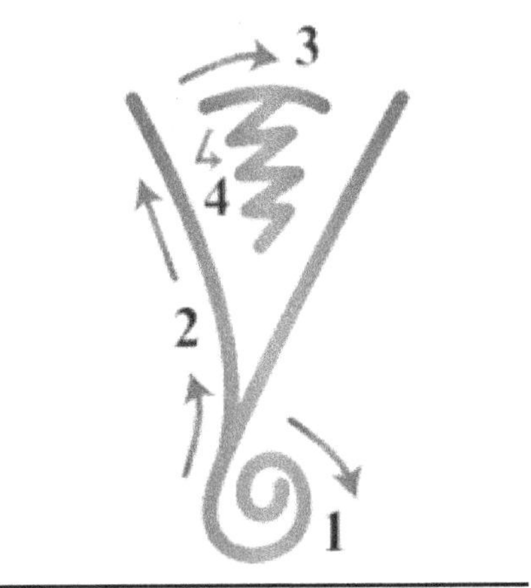

Dai Ko Mio-Tibetan Master Symbol

Dai Ko Mio (pronounced dee ko meo) is the symbol that reconnects to the Source, transforming at the spiritual level. Some RMT'S teach only one Master symbol, however I was taught both of them and use both of them. Dr. Usui did not teach this symbol. This symbol came from the Tibetan Usui system of Reiki.

The TFS works on all Chakras-past, present and future. The spirals help break up blockages and the entire symbol connects the three selves (Super-consciousness (Aumaukua),mind-consciousness(Uhane) and inner-self consciousness(Uni).

There is a difference of pronunciation between the two Master symbols. The first one is from Usui Ryoho Reiki and used by the Gakkai and Dr. Usui. This second symbol is sometimes taught alone and there is much contention that the first Master symbol Dai Ko Myo should always be used and taught if your particular RMT did not teach it. You should be attuned to this TFS also.

Also the Tibetan Fire Serpent enables the Kundalini to rise through the Chakra system. You may have heard this word from Yoga. Kundalini is Sanskrit for the energy that begins at the base of the spine and rises up in snake-like fashion through the Chakra system. It is a sacred energy. All the Chakras must be open for this sacred energy to rise up. This will bring change and healing. Reiki brings change. So, when you are working on the Client the Chakras will be cleared and by using the second Master TFS, you will be awakening the Kundalini. People may experience strong emotions. They may cry. Don't get upset; just be there for them and let them talk if they wish. The work you are doing is helping them to move forward.

The only person who can change you is you yourself. Reiki initiates the body to start its' own natural healing. Your mind and your body are very powerful. When you have received a treatment you should choose not to go back to the "old" way of thinking and doing. Reiki only initiates; it is totally up to you to complete the healing with your mind and your body. I always try to educate my Clients as to ways they can help themselves. Remember, this is not a miracle although I have seen people get extreme relief with just one session. There may be a need for on-going treatments and if the Client is also willing to do their own work for themselves; then they will attain their goal of being healed. At the very least, some relief should be achieved after each session.

I have given you the tools to use for yourself and your Clients. In tough cases, such as chronic disease, you may be stretched to your limit. Always ask for help from your RMT and your "Team" when you need it and don't have the experience to deal with whatever it is you are working on. As I said previously, there are also online groups who are willing to answer questions. Do the best you can. Loving intent is a powerful tool. Reiki too; especially with seven symbols, is also a very powerful gift from the Source. Adding the many modalities and tools also ramps up the energies. We never know for sure what exactly the Client may need so again, I repeat: use everything you have at your command. We also have to keep in mind "The Big Picture", meaning that before we come to Earth, we have chosen our lessons. The Client may have chosen the chronic disease as part of their learning on Earth. Be compassionate but remember you can't live their life. We are all in charge of our own path. I advise you to use all your gifts to the best of your ability and know that you have done what you needed to do for your Client.

TIBETAN FIRE SERPENT

This symbol awakens the Kundalini which allows the energy to rise up through each Chakra without releasing it from the Crown. Why would we want to do this?

The rising energy clears blockages and awakens energy in our body. We become connected to the Earth from the Root Chakra upwards throughout each Chakra.

The entire point of doing Reiki is to awaken the body's own healing energy. Our bodies do have the ability to heal us.

If you remember from the list we begin our Attunement with the Tibetan Fire Serpent in order to wake this energy. The Attunement places each symbol in the Aura.

The symbols are with you after the Attunements for the rest of your life. I believe that they awaken our body healing energy on an ongoing basis. However, using them on a consistent basis builds on this energy. You may notice after Attunements that you feel wonderful and many changes may come to you and in your life for the better. I do highly recommend getting and giving Attunements on a regular basis.

Tibetan Fire Serpent

(Page left blank to practice symbol)

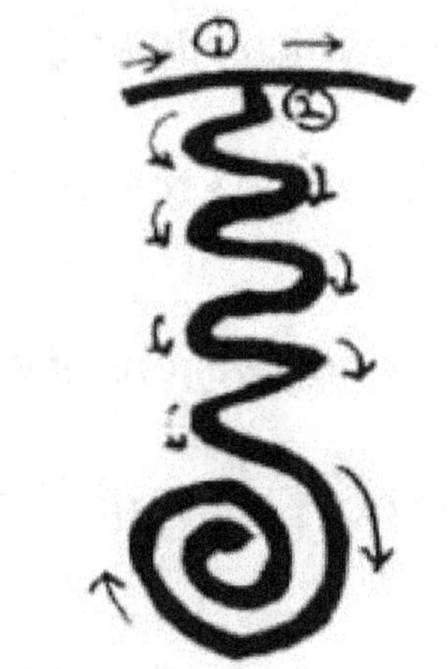

Universal

This symbol came to me in a dream or vision. The 5 tips of the star represent the 5 elements of the world we inhabit. The elements are the following: Earth, Air, Fire, Water and Spirit. The circle enclosing the star represents our world (which can be personal or general) and the forces contained therein. The bubbles on the outside represent our journey from one stage (ex.: birth) to the final stage which is when we cross over. The heart, of course represents Divine love as well as personal love and offers grounding for all the above. Also, the star represents God in Man. This is an all-inclusive symbol. I use it every time I do Reiki. The symbol chooses what level (either personal or general) that it will channel the energy to or perhaps both. I am very aware of the honor of this gift. I don't know why I was chosen to receive the symbol however; I know that others in different schools of Reiki have also received new symbols. You would place this at the end of the attunement. You may not choose to use this and it is up to your discretion. The other symbols are law, so to speak. You must use them to be effective. My thought is that once I begin teaching this symbol, it too will become law. I have been using it now for over five years and I have taught it to students of mine that have gone on to become Reiki Masters. This symbol has been a considerable blessing to me. I believe that as we grow into the Reiki light these new symbols are coming to us to make the energy we are using even more powerful. We need it!

Universal

(Page left blank to practice symbol)

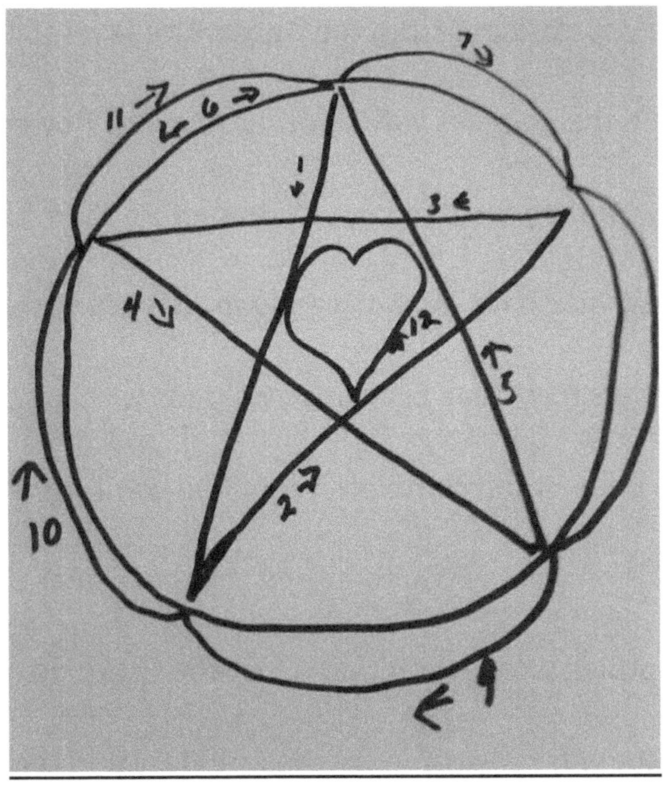

The Reiki Master should have integrity and discernment. Your intention is to share your knowledge and help your students grow into this work. At times you may not have taken your student from the Apprentice level to the Master level, they may have begun their classes with another teacher. However, do the best you can to impart what they need to know. I do require them to provide any Certification that they may have already received. My students attend classes as they desire at the levels they have previously paid for with me. I want them to really feel that they understand completely and feel comfortable. I differ in this aspect as most RMT's only allow you to attend that particular class that you have paid for. There is nothing wrong with that; I just choose to do my teaching a little differently. Some students only come for the one class and that is fine also. Only you can decide how to teach and what you are willing to extend to your student.

Most of this work will be learned by personal experience and your own personal research. These books and these classes are only the beginning. Another requirement that is an absolute must is: you must like people and you must have a lot of patience. Every person learns at their own level. That is one of the reasons why I allow them to come back as much as they wish to. Those who have the clear goal of becoming an RMT will benefit by assisting you in the classes and watching what you do. They cannot teach however, they can assist in other ways at your direction.

I always type up an outline for my classes enabling me to cover everything the student needs to know. This allows me to get my materials ready prior to the actual class. I hand out a lot of information along with the book of mine that is apropos to that particular class. As I am following the outline, I may decide to tweak it so the lesson will be more effective and it also helps to keep us on track timewise. I give the students a copy too so they will know what to expect. While you are teaching you also are always learning. I will include an example of an outline which you may wish to use for your classes. Feel free to change anything therein. What works for me as a teacher may not work for you. You can use these books as your manuals for teaching.

Class Outline for Level I

10:00	*Registration, Coffee, introductions & getting settled*
10:15	*Spiritual card for each, short discussion-Angels.*
10:30	*Introduction to teacher(s), Reiki, brief History, overview of materials & book.*
11:00	*Introduction to Chakras, chakra worksheet & discussion.*
11:15	*Introduction to Pendulum & dowsing.*
11:30	*Introduction to Aura & scanning by hand.*
11:45	*Grounding meditation (outside if possible)*
12-12:30	*Lunch (brown bag) coffee, tea & water available*
12:30	*Regroup, review, questions*
1:00	*Attunement discussion*
1:15	*Treatments – each student will learn about how to give/get a treatment including hand placements using the tools we have learned about.*
3:15	*Individual attunements-student receives this & Certification.*
4:00	*Certificate and payment.*

First level Reiki I

The student does not get a symbol in Level I. You should emphasize that most of the work will be done by them in their free time at home. My students can call me and I also try to have Reiki shares so they can get some practice and a treatment. Self-treatment is very important. It is absolutely vital to you.

The outline is what works for me in my classes. You are welcome to use it once you have reached Master Level (4) or tweak it in any way that works for you. I usually print up copies for everyone so we can all follow along.

I set up beforehand with all the handouts, the book, pen, notebook, a pack of 7 crystals for the Chakras, and a pendulum. I personally feel that the student will get much more out of the class if they have all the tools at hand. Some teachers advise students to get these things and that is ok too. I happen to enjoy sharing these tools with my students and they are included in my pricing.

I use the spiritual cards to determine where the participants in the class are on their particular path. Surprisingly, most classes are of like mind, meaning they are all about the same place in knowledge and experience with spiritual modalities. The cards are enjoyable but also note that you need to keep it brief. I also find that the meanings of each card are individual and also pertain to all the students. They also give the students an idea of what entities, such as Angels, are available for them to work with.

I do the Tree grounding meditation from my first book. I explain what grounding is and why we need it. We usually go outside if it is nice and bare feet to really connect with the earth energies and Universal energies.

There is a lot of information to share in these classes. Ultimately the brunt of the work will be done outside the class by the student. How much or what they do depends on how interested they are in progressing.

In Reiki Level II, we refresh from the previous class. I do the Guardian Angel meditation at some point. We spend quite a bit of time on the symbols because in order to get Certificate you must know them. I want to see you see, say and draw in the air, on paper and over the person you will be working on.

We also spend a lot of time doing treatments for each other. Each person will be guided from beginning to end of a full treatment. The list from my first book comes in handy to a new person because it details the treatment step-by-step. Use the lists for as long as you need to however, keep in mind that at some point you should be able to do this work without them (with the exception of the class outlines). Your diligence in practicing and studying will determine how effective a ***Reiki Alchemical Lightworker*** you will become! I know that you will be amazing when you are sharing this gift. Many blessings will flow from you to others and to you from others.

If you don't do that many treatments and/or classes; all these tools can be used to refresh yourself so you are effective at what you are focusing on. Focus on quality firstly and quantity secondly.

Outline for Level II Reiki

10:00	Coffee, Introductions, get settled
10:15	Angel Card
10:30	Brief review of Reiki Level I
10:45	Cho-Ku-Rei
11:00	Sei-Hei-Ki
11:15	Hon-Shah-Ze-Sho-Nen & review
12:00	Lunch
12:30	Meet your Guardian Angel Meditation
1:00	Treatments with each student participating On/off the table using symbols, crystals, auric scanning, pendulum, hand placement
3:00	Attunements for Level II & Certificate
4:00	Certificate and payment

Second Level Reiki

Usually but not always, the students take Reiki I and II in one weekend or over a two-day period. This is not my ideal because there is so much information to share but people are so busy it has to suffice. That is why I like to remain a resource and encourage the students to do the work on their own also.

Reiki II covers the symbols. You can learn them and internalize them in one day. Many have done it before you and many will continue to do so. I usually tell a little story for the HSZSN because it is long and it helps the student to remember each section of it. They also will have their own book and notebook with the symbols written down until they learn them by heart. We practice over and over until the student feels fairly comfortable with all of the symbols.

I then do the Guardian Angel meditation so each person has at least one Angel to work with if they haven't been working with Beings previously. Guardian Angels are instantly available when you make a request. This is an amazing resource. Sometimes they communicate with signs like feathers, or a line in a song. We can always ask questions in our minds and get an answer if we are open to the many ways in which Angels communicate.

We learn these things in the morning and in the afternoon we use our knowledge from both levels with all the symbols to do a treatment and receive one. I require my students to draw all the symbols on paper, in the air and over the person on the table without looking so I can see they have accomplished their goal.

They then receive their Attunement. At that same time we are using all the symbols and they are being placed in the students' Aura. It is my belief that once you have an Attunement, even if you are not using the Reiki on a regular basis, you are still deriving benefit on some microcosmic level.

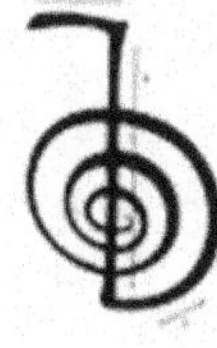

. This is the Cho-ku-rei which should be learned at Reiki II.

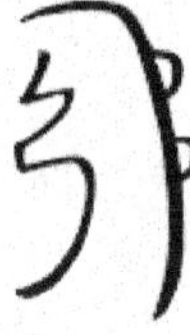

This is Sei-Hei-Ki also from Reiki II.

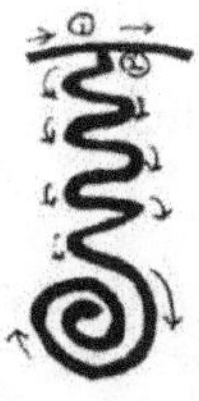

This is Tibetan Fire Serpent from Reiki II.

Class Outline for Adept or Master Level

10:00	*Meeting everyone, coffee and getting settled.*
10:30	*Ascended Master card or any card you like.*
10:45	*Going over requirements for RM/T and introducing concepts of Attunement, Hui Yin and Violet Breath. Practice!*
11:30	*Meditation to meet Reiki Guides*
12:00	*Lunch break*
12:30	*Attunements – we will be practicing these on each other knowing that we do not give them unless we are a RMT.*
1:30	*Antakharana and how to use it to make a Reiki grid or box.*
2:00	*Psychic surgery – with practice*
3:00	*Revisiting everything learned today, answering questions and discussing what we have learned. Treatment practice.*
	Adept level gets attunement adding Usui Master Symbol.
	RMT level gets attunement adding Tibetan Master & Universal.
4:00	*Certificate and payment.*

Reiki Master Teacher class outline

10:00	Intro, coffee & getting settled
10:15	Card
10:30	Refresher of previous 3 classes
11:30	Tibetan Master Symbol
12-12:30	lunch
12:30	Universal Master Symbol
1:00	Practice Attunement
1:30	Treatments using everything the student has learned
3:30	Student Attunement for all four levels
4:00	Certificate and payment.

Reiki Master Teacher

Once the student has become attuned to all four levels, I suggest that they perform a treatment in front of and with their RMT. Under a time constraint the student can do this during the treatment portion of the class as long as your RMT will allow that. If your RMT is willing, perhaps the student will be able to attend some treatments to observe and/or participate. Most students will not be doing treatments on a daily basis so that's where the lists come in and it is good to refresh your knowledge and skills prior to a treatment.

If you have a dedicated space for the Reiki treatment, you as the practitioner should clear with the pendulum, then see, say, draw the symbols directing them to all four corners which will cleanse the room and give your Team notice that you will be performing the treatment. Do you have to do this every time? I personally do however, I imagine that you can intend sending it on a continuous flow. This is where discernment enters. You make the decision as to what you will be doing. Also, as I have said-if you don't have a dedicated space just clear wherever you are in your mind or ask your "Team" to clear and do "band-aid" Reiki or a full treatment depending on the circumstances. You can use a bed, a chair or wherever you are able; depending on the circumstances. Also, for instance I draw the Cho-Ku-Rei over my home (in my mind) as a barrier from negative energies. You can also surround yourself, others, your home, your pets, or your car - with Light asking that only love be allowed to enter.

You can always ask for direction from the Angels and your Reiki guides. Quiet your mind, ask and you will receive thoughts or impressions of what to do. You can use your pendulum to ask Yes or No questions of your Angels and Guides.

Also, don't forget to journal your experiences. Write down everything-what worked, what happened, how the Client felt, what crystals used etc... you are building your own Alchemical Reiki formulae. I keep suggesting the journaling because as you use the Reiki and other modalities throughout the years, things can become confusing or forgotten. This allows you to have a record of what worked and what might not have. I especially like to journal certain dreams, visions, and any information I might obtain through a meditation. I go back over them periodically to refresh and also sometimes whatever happened may become clearer.

This is a lifelong journey. Please don't get intimidated. Go at your own pace and don't hesitate to ask for help if you need it. We are all working together in spirit.

As a Reiki Master please remain aware that your students are following your example. They look to you for integrity, help and guidance.

There are myriad ways to use Reiki. If you have a thought about the energy and wish to do it in another way that was not mentioned – go for it! We are only limited by our imaginations. Your sincere love and intention will allow the energy to channel through you to your Client.

With Reiki and the other tools you add, you will change yourself and the world for the highest good of all one person at a time! Welcome to the Team!

DOWSING

Dowsing was begun in my last book and I hope that you have continued to use this exceptionally helpful modality. Dowsing can be used to clear you, and other people, homes, cars –whatever you feel needs to be cleared. Dowsing can also shield all the aforementioned. How would you go about this? You would have your pendulum in hand and ask to clear (whatever you are working on) and once the pendulum indicates this is done; then I would ask for shielding and the pendulum will spin until that has been completed. Dowsing picks up on energies from the earth. Remember I told you previously that everything in the Universe is vibrating? Dowsing utilizes these vibrations to do what you have directed it to do.

Most of my students have so much fun learning and using their pendulum. They carry it with them wherever they go and use it as needed. You can dowse food, vitamins that you may need, herbs and anything along those lines. Also, bless and thank your food with Reiki.

I am including a guide on the next page which I received from Tyhson Banighan, Master Dowser and Illuminator. You can tweak the wording if you wish to work for someone else but remember we must always ask permission and use it for the highest good of all concerned.

Guide to Assist Healing using Pendulum

THE EXTRAORDINARY HEALING ARTS ACADEMY

Host of the Wellness show on Facebook

Contact: www.tyhsonbanighen.ca or tyhson@me.com.

The deep clearing protocol (long form) is used to strengthen your bioenergy field to exclude intrusions into your field by outside forces such as: entities, manmade energy interrupters such as cell phone towers, smart meters, microwave or scalar waves etc. also: inside forces such as: unresolved trauma issues such as toxic emotions, core fractures etc.

To obtain a copy go to: https://rebrand.ly/41lx4.

Deep clearing Short Clearing Statement – Fill in or enter what you want to clear within the brackets.

Spin your pendulum counterclockwise while state the short clearing statement below:

I (state your birth name) in my Holy Name translate, transmute, transfigure, heal and repair all non-beneficial energies, core fractures and toxic emotions related to: (any limited beliefs from childhood or whatever). I ask for the assistance of (Lakshmi, God or Goddess or Light Team) to undertake this clearing throughout my matriarchal and patriarchal families of origin, soul family and star family lineages and throughout the multi-dimensional levels of my beings, all timelines-past, present and future, and all space-time continuums and dimensions both known or unknown. I love you. I am sorry. Please forgive me. In my Holy Name I declare it so. So be it. It is done. Thank you.

Deep clearing Short Clearing Manifestation Statement.

Spin your pendulum clockwise and state words to this effect:

I am a whole sovereign human being free of any and all intrusions into my energy from any and all sources known or unknown. I always have been and always will be loved by the Creator no matter what I think I may have done wrong. I am always guided by the Creator to be in the right place at the right time and therefore, I am always safe and secure. I remember why I incarnated and what unique gifts I have to deliver to the world. In my Holy Name I declare it so. So be it. It is done. Thank you.

You should plan on doing this until you feel it is finished. This is a long-term

Commitment because it took years for your body to develop into what it is today.

Our bodies regenerate our cells every seven years so it is possible with intent and work to change the dis-ease you may be experiencing.

There are many facets to dowsing to do with healing. The (ASD) American Society of Dowsers can help with this and there is a very good Facebook group where they shared this healing tool. Tyler Brannighan leads that group. Dowsing taps into energies from Gaia (Mother Earth) as I said. There are energy lines, vortexes and energy sinks. You are already using the pendulum to diagnose the Chakra system. You are also using it to clear and shield. This too, is a lifelong study. There is so much knowledge that we will never be able to encompass it all in our work. Use what resonates with you and works effectively for you and your Client.

Dowsing can especially be used to remove negative entities and blockages. You may ask your pendulum any yes or no question. You will receive an answer.

I have these sayings on my altar and use them every day. However you use it is up to you. You have all the tools now to become a successful Reiki Master Teacher. I wish you many blessings on your path to learning how to help yourself and others. This is deep healing on an extraordinary level. As a RMT it is up to your discretion as to what tools you will use in your ***Alchemical Reiki Lightworker formula.***

We cannot always know at what level we are effecting a change. It may take time for some of the tools to work for your Client. Do not get discouraged. Remember you as the RMT step outside of time and space to do your work. We can become overwhelmed when we realize that every single person on Earth needs help for something. We can only do our best, one person at a time. Also, keep working on yourself because this is beneficial on all levels. By working on yourself, you also learn what works and what may not.

Dowsing is an extremely helpful tool. I find it fascinating. There is so much to learn from any modality that you incorporate into your work that it seems we will never know everything. That is ok! Whatever we do know, use and expand will generate healing on some level.

I encourage you to go forth with your knowledge and formulae! You don't need to have a business in order to help others. You are an ***Alchemical Reiki Lightworker!***

About the Author

Linda came to this work after the death of her husband. She had a paranormal experience with him and decided there had to be more to this life than what we have been told which initiated her spiritual journey where she learned Reiki, HUNA, Crystals, Angels, Dowsing just to name a few. Shamanistic thought allows her to step outside Time/Space to do the most effective work possible for her Clients.

She lives in upstate NY with her fiancée and two rescue cats. She loves Reiki, reading, writing, travel, nature, boating, gardening and her family.

alchemyofreiki.com is her website and if you'd like to get in touch you can email: spiritedlinda@alchemyofreiki.com. Follow her on Twitter, Facebook, Instagram.

If you enjoyed the book(s) please do leave a review on Amazon or Goodreads and thanks! I am honored that you chose to read my book (s)!

www.ingramcontent.com/pod-product-compliance
Lightning Source LLC
Chambersburg PA
CBHW081315250726
48662CB00008B/2581

* 9 7 8 1 6 8 6 1 0 7 1 3 9 *